I0765815

DISCLAIMER AND TERMS OF USE AGREEMENT:

(Please Read This Before Using This Report)

This information is not presented by a medical practitioner and is for educational and informational purposes only. The content is not intended to be a substitute for professional medical advice, diagnosis, or treatment. Always seek the advice of your physician or other qualified health provider with any questions you may have regarding a medical condition. Never disregard professional medical advice or delay in seeking it because of something you have read.

Since natural and/or dietary supplements are not FDA approved, they must be accompanied by a two-part disclaimer on the product label: that the statement has not been evaluated by FDA and that the product is not intended to "diagnose, treat, cure or prevent any disease.

The author and publisher of this course and the accompanying materials have used their best efforts in preparing this course. The author and publisher make no representation or warranties with respect to the accuracy, applicability, fitness, or completeness of the contents of this course. The information contained in this course is strictly for educational purposes. Therefore, if you wish to apply ideas contained in this course, you are taking full responsibility for your actions.

The author and publisher disclaim any warranties (express or implied), merchantability, or fitness for any particular purpose. The author and publisher shall in no event be held liable to any party for any direct, indirect, punitive, special, incidental or other consequential damages arising directly or indirectly from any use of this material, which is provided "as is", and without warranties.

As always, the advice of a competent legal, tax, accounting, medical or other professional should be sought. The author and publisher do not warrant the performance, effectiveness or applicability of any sites listed or linked to in this course.

All links are for information purposes only and are not warranted for content, accuracy or any other implied or explicit purpose.

Contents

<u>Combating Stress Through Massage Therapy</u>

There may be many remedies for relieving stress and tension, which are hard to avoid in the complexities of modern life for any age-group, but among the most enjoyable and peaceable ones is opting for massage therapy.

Medical research has pointed out that most of today's health problems are due to stress, which can be caused also from improper diets, following an unhealthy life style, working overtime or in a disorganized way etc. The common factor among all these possible causes for stress is that no matter what the source of the stress, it has a damaging effect on the bodily systems, which are needed to be maintained properly for sustained, healthy output.

This is why it is important to banish stress and the eliminate the factors that lead to it; if this is not possible immediately and needs to be worked slowly at, the best way out is to take up a proven stress-relieving treatments, such as massage therapy affords in order to combat various health issues that can crop up due to uncontrolled stress. These include gastrointestinal disorders, cardiac disease, loss of memory besides decreased immune function.

Of course, there is always medication for relieving stress and while pill-popping is popular and even advertised highly on the TV, it is not recommended as either a long-term or even a safe option. This is why massage therapy has gained so much importance in recent times with people having experienced first-hand the benefits and the joys of a good, therapeutic massage and with so many forms of massage abounding, not to mention massage parlors and literature promoting the practice, is it a surprise that it is such a favorite topic?

Not really would be the right answer – for there are so many people in the world who have benefited from a good, timely and warm massage therapy and the thoughtful manipulation of body tissues that relax mind, body, muscle, sinew, nerves and much more – releasing not only muscular tension and metabolic waste, but also promoting nutrient delivery for hastening tissue-healing tissue.

Thus, the current belief that massage therapy is a boon is not far-off because its blessings are a-plenty for those that have tried it and come out significantly more at peace, in better health – both physically and mentally and better equipped also to face the demands of a changing world.

Massage Therapy For Complete Body Relaxation

From the realm of alternate medicine and healthcare systems that were centuries old, such as those practiced in India, Japan, Sweden and China come the best forms of massage therapy that are aimed at preventing, controlling and even curing chronic ailments so the individual can enjoy an enhanced sense of holistic healing.

What makes massage therapy such a blessing for modern, stress-filled lives and people is the fact that it works on varied principles that boost our body's immune system, helps release harmful chemicals from the body and has a joyful effect of peace, contentment and relaxation due to a trained therapist's hands working to improve health by acting directly on the muscular, nervous, circulatory and immune systems at one time.

Massage therapy basically releases endocrine (the happy hormones) and combines comprehensive knowledge of human anatomy, specific body part healing techniques, pathology and human psychology so is only beneficial when performed by a trained therapist who has received proper education in all these aspects – learn about the credentials to become one, or even to pick one!

National Standards For Massage Therapy Certification

So far, there is only one standard that is nationally recognized for massage therapy certificate, which is controlled by the NCBTMB, the abbreviation of National Certification Board for Therapeutic Massage and Bodywork. Any massage therapy services who apply for the national certificates will be evaluated and if their service reflects a good standard, NCBTMB will give them a certificate that is recognized nationally.

The Identity of The National Certification Board for Therapeutic Massage And Bodywork

The NCBTMB is founded by the American Massage Therapy Association (AMTA). AMTA itself founded NCBTMB in 1992 because of the need to set standards for massage therapy services that could be found easily at that time everywhere. Furthermore, at that time, massage therapy was gaining its popularity and many people were attracted by the service. A certificate was therefore very important to determine which services were recommended and which services had to improve on their quality. Today, the NCBTMB certification is still held high, and its role is not just to declare the quality of massage therapy services. It now acts also as a license in most states for massage therapy services before they can start operating, so it has become a must for massage therapy services to own their own national certificates.

Requirements For The Massage Therapy Certification

Of course the application for this national massage therapy service certification is not as easy as it seems. Applicants must meet certain requirements in order to get the NCBTMB massage therapy service certification. These requirements are stated by the National Certification Board for Therapeutic Massage and Bodywork itself.

The certificant must :

1. Finish stipulated levels of massage therapy education
2. Submit evidence of training
3. Get and submit evidence of one's experience
4. Demonstrate excellent core massage therapy abilities

5. Demonstrate understanding of the field, comprising of practical comprehension and knowledge of fair commerce practice
7. Pass a tough written examination

These are requirements only for initial certification. In addition to them, the status of the certificants must be renewed every four years. Applicants must also show evidence of work experience in massage therapy and proof of finishing the massage therapy education upon renewal.

The True Meaning of NCBTMB Certification

There are actually numerous functions of NCBTMB massage therapy certification, such as acting as license in some states. However, its most crucial function is to protect the employers, therapists, and the public.

NCBTMB massage therapy service certification also ensures the consistency of high quality provided by massage therapy services. All massage therapists who bear the status of "Nationally Certified in Therapeutic Massage and Bodywork" must promise that they will continue their professionalism. Hence, NCBTMB massage therapy certification identifies massage therapists that the clients can count on.

<u>Massage Therapy Today</u>

Modern world need modern methods of relaxation. Clinically speaking nowadays hospitals and spa partners introduce the new innovation that is massage therapy. This reading will shed some light to the reads about therapeutic massage.

It was the Chinese who pioneered massage therapy. It was them who also introduced it in the modern times. The main function of this is to help ease the pain and it was a form of relaxation for them. Sometimes it is used by medical experts as a healing process applied for some illnesses.

These are helpful information that will aid you in understand the true concept behind therapeutic massage.

Massage Therapy is a modern technique to help improve various health problems and is used to calm the nerves down. It is also called a healing power. In China 3,000 years pass our times, massage became an aborigin of culture to them. It was practiced as a part of their medical technique of curing the physical aspect of their wellbeing.

Because of the importance of therapeutic massage, it became a solution and ritual to those people who wants to stay healthy and relax. Often, nowadays even medical evaluation says that massage therapy is a solution to some patients, for instance stroke victims and other victims of muscle depletion sickness. This is done as a daily routine to ensure people its full benefits which this process is a great help on. It is no longer called "old method of medication." As the passing of time, it became popular and it is now favored by the public.

This method, in general, includes rubbing and manipulation on the affected areas or as a whole. It can be applied to any part of the body as needed to lessen the intensity of pain and cure tightness of muscles due to stress and tension of daily work.

The basic techniques of massage therapy:

Touching hard muscles, ligaments, soft tissues and even joints.

Massage Therapy For Complete Body Relaxation

Exercising hard muscles in order to control tightening.
Used as touch therapy for babies and used to soften muscles
Soft touching
Kneading the muscles
Touching or soft thumping
Using electric tense
Spasm relaxation
Ultra sound machine with gel for deep penetration

Application used in various ways, composing of more than 250 kinds of massage therapy. Therapists call these in different styles, like Swedish Massage, Reflexology, Touch Therapy, Somatic Acupressure, Sports Massage and Neuromuscular Massage. These are therapists who concentrate in one kind of massage. In some hospitals massage varies in modalities depending on the damaged area of the body. Physical therapists schedule patients on how often the application of massage is to be done. It is a case-to-case basis until such time the patient fully recovers.

The products used by massage therapist varies from different kinds of clients. They should have the bed, table, powder, lotion or oil. But most of them use aroma therapy as stimulating massage oil.

Massage contributes a big factor to ones health. However it also depends on how well the physical application is being given to the client. Sporty people usually injures their feet while engaging on their game. Some are due to various illnesses and others from physical stress. Some medical experts prefer to recommend massage therapy in replacement of oral medication. It contributes a big factor to society. Plenty of experienced therapists grows more and more. Modern times conclude that it is meant only for relaxation. However it is also a great help to those who have illnesses and injury since it will lessen oral intake of pills. In some cases it is also being recommended as weight management program.

The Basics Of The Massage Therapy Licensure Program

To be a good physical Therapist one should undergo training after graduation and should pass the licensure examination. Not only in Columbia but also in the U.S. on their 37 states practices the same law. To practice your profession as a therapist, it is a requirement that you should be license to let people know that you are qualified to that position. In addition to this, most states required applicants for the job as medical or physical therapist a long training program in order conduct business with their patients or customers.

Massage therapy is sometimes called oral replacement of medication. It is one way of healing and getting rid of stress, mentally and physically. Nowadays, people are well   informed about the good effects of massaging the body to obtain good health. It is also a physiological treatment to replace any form of medication to those who are ill and weak. They should be a license therapist to assure the public that they are capable of handling them physically and the exact reflexivity of the body. This will make them credible to practice with legal back-up.

Requirements to be a Massage Therapist:

The U.S. government requires all therapists to take the licensure examination. Some places do not require, and they practice it in a small town, city, or country. Local governments have their own requirements that have the same connection with other countries. Students should not allow themselves to practice their profession as a massage therapist without license in order to work legally and regularly in other countries. This is to protect themselves that their patients for any future dispute. A good license can make a practitioner the best bet to as safe massage therapy.

State Requirements for Students:

- He or she should complete the required number of formal classes in massage therapy program.
- You should pass all national and state board examination.
- Students should continue further studies in order to have license.

Aspects of Good quality Massage Therapy Program

Students should consider a certain aspects and should know how massage therapy licensure program is being chosen.

The first thing to know is what kind of licensure program thus your state has. Around 1300 programs, about 300 are only accepted by a state board officials or the Department of Education.
State or Professional certification Board for licensure doesn't accept more than two-third of the program due to some reasons. Choose a program with proper accreditations. That way you are sure to get a genuine license. There are fake schools that offer students tuitions for less amount of money. But, they are bogus and should not be taken seriously. Make sure to research on the kind of reputation those schools have. This can make you realize that it is worth paying the right amount of money to ensure an authentic license.

Licensing programs are different in every school. They can be a bit confusing. To make certain what choice of curriculum to take, know your interests. Then in know will come a very well planed out decision. Stringing a balance between your interests and what is needed as requirements by the NCBTMB. This department is responsible for giving licenses to students who meet the necessary requirements.

Studying is always a good way to better life. Knowing what to study on to succeed is a start.

Massage Schools

This is to inform aspiring student on the many things the Northwestern school has to offer of future massage therapists. Included are schedules and benefits that can be gained in enrolling into their courses.

Students who have an excellent rating in school seek a place to enroll to have a god perspective in life. They prefer to stay in Northwestern's school of therapeutic massage. It started to accept qualified students. The school provides awareness program to all the students so that people will have an idea of the importance of massage in their health.. Physiologists suggest to their patients on how massage contribute to their lives and recommend a session for early of recoveries to maintain god health and minimize expenditures by asking aid from a therapist.

Northwestern school teaches their students on how to manage pain and how they will go to communicate with their clients. As part of health care they ensure their patients about wellness and health status of everyone. They are being taught on how to contribute and participate in our daily routine. Students undergo orientation about patients pain and to promote close relationship with their clients and to the community itself.

A thirty-six semester credit with sessions of 780 hrs. give students a good learning over major science the school has 340 hours of personal laboratory teaching and share some medical experience inside the learning institute of massage therapy teaching clinic and some surrounding the school accepts and intellectual professors and some social oriented people, plus mostly some of the in demand therapist in Minnesota.

The school building has two 1100 square feet area for laboratory. It is composed of one table for massage for every pair of students, they usually hold their lecture anywhere within the school campus. The location of the school is in Burnsville Natural Care Center. They are open on all Mondays, Wednesdays, Fridays and Saturdays.

For those who intend to enroll evening classes and weekend studies, they are allowed to attend on Tuesdays, Wednesdays and Thursday nights. If you wish to attend a full-time class once in a

Massage Therapy For Complete Body Relaxation

while, you can have it on Saturdays. They offer two choices of sessions. You can either take it in the morning of in the afternoon during Mondays, Wednesdays, Fridays and Saturdays. New enrollees are being accepted in the beginning of the year January, mid-year in May and lastly in September. It take for about 12 months to finish the syllabus of the course. So, depending on which month a students enrolls that's the basis for finishing the course. Those mentioned earlier are enrolment schedules of the day classes.

The students are required to attend 780 hours of classes in order to fully understand the different parts of the human anatomy. 195 hours of Physiology, Anatomy, Path physiology, Kinesiology, and Nutrition. Minnesota has the largest capacity of program in massage therapy itself. They limit their students to a small quantity because they want to make sure that they can efficiently teach them well. Their name is known throughout the other states in the massage institutions community. This is on account of their well established instructors who are certified. These professors are eager to help the next line of massage therapists to carry-on the legacy with pride. Their devotion for their work stands out in everyway knowing that their students are also willing to take on the challenges that lies ahead.

Wide-ranging studies that are handled by outstanding practitioners are the key to getting the best education in any field of expertise a student has a passion to study in is what this school has to offer. Practicum are essential in preparation for making sure that students are well practices with performing hands-on tasks. The school includes ample amounts of time for them to enhance their skills. As they begin to grow more comfortable with using their knowledge and transforming it into their own, they become better.

Those are the many amenities that this school has to offer. So, if in the future you are contemplating on getting a good degree on therapeutic massage, this school is for you!

<u>Choosing The Best Massage Therapy School</u>

There is an ever growing need of enrollees to enter into the best massage schools in their area. Helping them to make their choice meet the criteria they will use in the future is this article.

The growth of the spa industry and wellness centers have sprung a new hype of getting a degree on massage therapy schools. Its popularity is now overwhelming that entering into the best school is the main agenda most students are looking for.

This is why qualifying for a first-class and well recognized institute for therapists remains to be on the top list. A good curriculum is one basis. The facilities of the school is another. The most important factor that needs to be looked into is qualification of the course that meet the requirements of the certification and regulatory board.

There are many aspects of therapeutic massage that have course on. If your are planning to enter this kind of career, then know which specialization is the first step you need to take. Zoom-in on the field that makes you enthralled the most. This will keep you from changing your mind in the future. Various examples would include therapeutic massages for sports injuries, massages for pediatrics or geriatrics and some are for relaxation or luxury massages. There are other forms and applications for therapeutic massages that are needed by people or patients. That's why it is quite imperative to get a closer look into your preference. This will make sure you're specialization will get you a job where you're needed. On the one hand, if you are still not sure of which path to take go to an institution that offers a broader lessons on massage therapy techniques. This will keep the employment window wide open for you.

The reality about getting your license as a massage therapist is sadly dependent on the requirements that national state regulatory board has issued. There is no unified requirements that can become basis for your certification. They vary from one state to another. This might be a good indication for choosing the right school for you. List the requirements for licensure in your state. Then as soon as you do that go ahead and basing on your information at hand, select and qualify the schools that meet the requirement. If their curriculum is design according to the state licensure program then you're assured to pass the requirements to become certified.

Massage Therapy For Complete Body Relaxation

Among other things, further and thorough investigation must be done to make sure you are making the right choice. Accreditation of the school programs are focal points in searching for strength of the school. A good reputation that precedes it and highly-qualified professors make a powerful combination that superior schools. What out for these indicators and you'll never go wrong.

Rediscovering The Wonders Of Massage

Due to hectic schedules and busy lifestyle people tend to feel devastated and tired physically, mentally and emotionally. Stress sometimes lead to a weak heart, and uncontrolled sugar that makes you a diabetic person and a stroke victim.

Soft human touch can remove stress in our lives. With this underlying fact, people get interested and plan to venture in spa business discovering the miracle result of body and foot massage. Total relaxation improves one's health and social lifestyle. Foreign visitors usually enjoy a body, facial or foot massage offered in hotels and tourist spots for their reasonable prices.

Spending extra money cannot do any harm in your budget. It is very useful and anybody is entitled to pamper oneself and enjoy a good day off by having a massage at any spa parlor.

Going in a spa center once or twice a week will not destroy your schedule. It would even make you feel relaxed and let you enjoy every minute of the massage session.

Body Rub 101

Secure the place you want to be. It should be warm and comfortable to both of you and your companion. Avoid contact with the outside world in order to give enough time to observe the condition and location. It should be warm and welcoming. Drapes will be suitable and air conditioned room will give you a much better feeling. It is advised to take a hot shower before starting the pleasure of body massage. It should start at the head to feel relaxed. Chinese scented candles or any flavored scent will help a lot by stimulating the olfactory nerves. It is advisable to let your partner choose whether to use oil, lotion or a mixture of both in order to create a smooth sensation on your body.

Resorts are the best places to find time to relax. A simple drape of white satin and clean sheets will add to the subtle feeling of inner peace. You may try lying flat on the bed, smelling the sea breeze, and feeling the touch of your partner. This can release all the muscle pain and stress. Ballad and love songs can create a feeling of happiness and fulfillment while enjoying your partners hand touching your whole body. It is also recommended that sometimes it is

Massage Therapy For Complete Body Relaxation

adventurous to take a vacation at resorts and so the session while smelling the fresh air and lying flat on the sand.

Be clean physically. Sanitation is very important by checking all the facilities and your partner as well. It is necessary to examine the hands for long finger nails that would be a cause of scratching your skin. The sheets should be clean and should smell good. A hard surface is advisable for you to lie down. Nerve endings should be touched as well to give pleasure and contentment during massage session. Good touch of hands will create a good experience and an unforgettable memory.

Give total consideration for the whole time while having a massage. It helps stimulate blood and regulate air pressure to your body. Tell your companion about how to enjoy the session. Appreciate anything your partner is doing to build a good relationship. Try to relax yourself although some people have the potential of taming your emotions. Feel each touch.

Experience the good effect of massage for yourself and you will notice that you will plan to have another session next time around. Your mind and body has an instinctive reaction to every sensitive matter since it creates a good result and activates all your senses. That's the way you do it. Body massage is a great experience and very memorable. It will enhance you to have a different lifestyle. Start early and be proud of yourself.

Intimacy is often lost in the world of handy phones and internets. That is why the need to be close to a partner is very important. This will help the wellness of the whole being of intact. Allow the experience to take over and you will soon know how it feels to be pampered again.

Massage Therapy Continuing Education

Massage therapy is not only about learning how to rub someone up the right way - it requires one to enroll and successfully complete nationally recognized certifications courses to be a trained as a masseuse or masseur

Modern lifestyles have added stress even as they have made so many advancements for people of today, which is why apart from the regular needs of medical healthcare professionals who recommend physiotherapy for patients in need of muscular pain relief; there are several thousands of people who go in for massage therapy for their general well being. This is the reason why massage therapy experts are so much in demand today, but they do need much more than a passing knowledge of the human anatomy and a healing touch; they need a continuing education plan to maintain a career in massage therapy, which may be required by state law as in the case in the US.

This mainly includes having access to the American Massage Therapy Association (which is the most important governing body for this field of work) as a qualified member and obtaining a certification from NCBTMB (or, the National Certification Board for Therapeutic Massage and Bodywork). Besides these qualifications, a trained massage expert also needs to regularly update training as expected by the National standards governing Massage Therapy Continuing Education Panels of their state/country.

At times, the regulatory requirements for massage therapists differ from state to state in the US with nearly 13 states only applying certain local ordinances for these experts and the way they are to function; but, for students keen to take up this work as a career option, it is important to gain knowledge beyond local requirements so they can practice legally in other states if so desired, for better career prospects.

This is why gaining comprehensive knowledge about the pursuing added qualifications for a massage therapist is important for students who are serious about being recognized as professionals on a national basis.

For example, 37 states and the District of Columbia have a common standard for licensure laid down by the AMTA (American Massage Therapy Association), which is a form of the NCBTMB

Massage Therapy For Complete Body Relaxation

certification and therapists wishing to practice in these states need to have an education guided by this body's format to be qualified to practice anywhere in the continent.

Some of these continuing education needs put down by the AMTA include students needing to put in a minimum of 48 hours of massage therapy every 4 years as continuing education, beginning with their 1st full year that they hold a Professional Active Membership in this body; other programs they join must fulfill the specifications of the AMTA or have NCBTMB approval to be considered legal besides actual and experiential trainings as well as theory training and research!

After the completion of their coursework that fits under the above criterion, the student-therapists must submit proof they have worked in this field of continuing education and also renew their membership every 4 years (an AMTA requirement, which can be done by filling up a form online)

So, renew the interest in a massage therapy career that is bound to flourish with the way the world is turning to alternate forms of healing today - and go for it!

<u>Starting A Mobile Massage Therapy Business</u>

Massage therapy is increasing being looked upon as a lucrative career option by many people with a healing hand and knowledge of the techniques of specialized massage therapy forms, so a mobile therapy unit is a great way to begin small and reap big dividends – through careful planning!

Not only has the modern lifestyle provided for growth, career fulfillment, entrepreneurship and advancements in every sphere of life but it has also provided for more stress to perform well and thus increased the value of alternate healing techniques, such as massage therapy! It is not wonder then that what used to be chiefly considered a physiotherapist's domain is now so much in demand as a value-added service in parlors, spas, health farms and even hotels as people crave rest, relaxation and peacefulness that a good massage therapist can provide with a flick of the wrist and spin of the fingers!

While it may not always be possible to rent out large and grand looking offices or commercial chambers for a massage therapy business, one can start small with the venture of providing quality massages at affordable costs by investing in a van so as to offer mobile massage therapy packages.

It is also a considerable lower investment than renting or buying a place and employing many people with added overheads; besides, having a mobile massage therapy business allows one to decide schedules according to their convenience, have more than one location to operate from and thus wider reach to customers, they are self-employed and enjoy more freedom than massage therapists working in a parlor under a boss and can also thus be totally independent in setting regulations for work as they please and deem fit.

Investing in a movable massage therapy business also reduces the expenses related to a regular set-up in an office environment besides eliminating much of the equipment one would require to fill space or even the salary of a receptionist and manager as such; other headaches such as property insurance and utility costs are also considerably reduced in a mobile unit.

Massage Therapy For Complete Body Relaxation

With the small private area afforded by a mobile massage unit, there is the added attraction of therapists being able to offer couple-massages that are a sensual treat for many partners who cannot enjoy the togetherness of such an experience at a parlor in quite the same way besides a mobile unit allows the entrepreneur to visit home-bound clients and those with a disability just as well. Even those with a time-limitation can be attended to in the privacy of the mobile massage unit with the therapist making the appointment somewhere near the client's office/home.

However, with all these heavy advantages to a mobile business as a massage therapist, there are equal number of downsides, which include taking care of self employment taxes that are typically more; having to take care of health and vehicle insurance on your own, incurring more fuel and maintenance cost for the automobile, extra commuting long-term, physical tiredness and mental strain of dealing with varied client demands at odd hours besides having to take care of advertising your services and business developments.

Weight the pros and cons of the decision and choose wisely if you are cut out for making it in the mobile massage therapy business – after all, nobody knows your needs better than you!

<u>Massage Therapy Products</u>

There are different kinds of massage products being used by the physical therapist. It lies on how the person applies such product. Know them up-close in this article.

Usually, oils and lotions are being mixed with powder to soothe one's skin. Products being used by therapist varies on what kind of massage session they are going to apply. Each product has its usage. Mostly in spa parlors they choose to use massage oil or they adhere to the client's preference. Mainly achieving the best kneading the body necessitates must be met by the masseuse.

Massaging with oil

The use of massage oil contributes a good effect to both massage therapist and the client. It slides easily and it is being absorbed by the skin. All kinds of massage oil are admired by people. Even baby oil being applied on the newborn makes the mother confident about using touch therapy to help the baby's development faster. When moms lovingly caress their young ones the child feel a sense of security.

Some therapist prefers to use stimulating massage oil with natural refreshing blend of citrus products. There are plenty of essential oil new Ferri, Tangerine, Peppermint, Almond oil, Citrus oil, grape oil, Sesame oil, Avocado oil, and many more. Any form of essential oil is applicable to one's body and its safe and refreshing. There's also what they call the holy oil that is derived from essential which is absorb by the tissues. Most essential oils have an aroma therapy smell that penetrates to our senses. These types of oil sometimes help soothe dry skin and helps improve the condition of the skin by making it look healthier when being applied after taking a shower.

It provides natural response to our reflexes; minimize tension and releases stress due to physical fatigue and daily anxiety. It helps and make the body feel more calm and at ease. One feels good and for some drift away slowly into sleep. Right after a tension relieving massage all the muscles are loosen up that even insomniacs can't resist the calling of their beds.

Massaging with lotion

Massage Therapy For Complete Body Relaxation

Lotions are alternative means if oil is not available. But there are people who prefer to use lotion because of Vitamin E that are present in that product. It softens the skin and the smell lasts longer on it. It also moisturizes dry skin cells and helps restore dullness that is present in the body. Also an anti-aging agent it replaces your skin's dead cells using anti-oxidant agents. Some countries have more highly advanced skin therapy applications than others. But the use of lotions as one of the best products for massages will never be outdated.

Everyone needs to be treated like a baby once in a while. It can rejuvenate the whole mindset allowing for more high spirits. When the body is eases out of tension it can be more productive. Rebuilding a proper attitude to go back into the word and conquer it. The much needed rest coupled with euphoric oil or lotion massage will surely make anyone feel like they are being reborn. The uses of these different products add more variations and excitement to the whole massage experience. They can stimulate the senses when just the right pressures are applied to the exact points.

How To Choose Massage Therapy Tables

Besides professional skills in massaging, a massage therapy table is also required for massaging business. There are many factors that will determine which massage therapy tables are suitable for the massaging business and, therefore, massage therapists have to be careful in selecting the right equipment for their business.

The first factor that massage therapists have to take into account is whether they need a movable or a stationary massage therapy table. This depends on their type of business and the space that they have. For example, if you want to give massaging service not only in your office, but to your clients' homes, a portable table is a must for you. A portable massage therapy table also has **a number of benefits compared to a stationary one**. Some of them are :

- They are cheaper in terms of cost
- You can bring the table easily to your clients' places to satisfy them
- When you want to re-arrange your things, it will be easier to move the table
- You can use it for dual-practice (both in-office and mobile services)

On the other side of the coin, a stationary table is also a good choice for those who want to specialize in in-office service only. It also provides more stability and is stronger than the portable one. Generally, stationary massage therapy tables are more expensive than portable ones.

Guidelines in Buying Massage Therapy Tables

Apart from the movable or non-movable type, there are other factors which you have to pay close attention to before purchasing massage therapy tables. The factors are :

- Weight and stability
- Durability
- Density or firmness of coverings
- Surface durability
- Vulnerability to chemical mixture such as lotions or oils
- Availability of extra add-ons

Massage Therapy For Complete Body Relaxation

- Ease to be cleaned

Besides that, there are also individual factors such as the affordability and the type of business that you will run. You can also purchase a simple one and then, in the future, you can further embellish it with new add-ons or upgrade the table. The objective of this is to boost the comfort and also give the clients a whole new experience while they are massaged.

There are also **various accessories** that you can buy to equip your massaging tables. They are:

- Adjustable rests for head, feet and arms
- Bolsters
- Face holes
- Cushions
- Headsets
- Pregnancy accommodations
- Carrying case
- Warmers

Warranties is also an important factor to consider. You would not want to spend a lot of money on a table and then you had to spend another large sum of money because it is broken, right?

It is imperative to consider these accessories and different types of massage therapy table before purchasing one. It ensures that you have made the right choice by choosing the right table so that you will not regret buying it in the future. With the right massage therapy table, your business will keep improving and the clients will all be satisfied.

<u>Massage Table – Tips On Picking The Perfect One!</u>

It is widely recognized as a form of relieving stress, inducing sleep and helping tired muscles relax – yes, we are talking about a massage! But, for a massage to be all this, the perfect massage table is very important; so, here are some useful tips on choosing the best massage table!

It may be that you are taken in by the number of fabulous designs massage tables are now available in, but it is advisable to wait and compare these for quality and pricing against others existing in the growing market so your back massage is more soothing than ever!

Look for the basics of a massage table along the concepts that make it a dependable and worthy proposition to invest in for your good health: check out various designs, type of construction, comfort and firmness factors besides the weight (both of the table and on your pocket!)

A good massage table needs to be not only good to look at, but functional and practical as well for your added ease of transportation; choose one that is portable and made of good quality, whatever your budget.

Check out various parts of the massage table that takes your fancy and look for design details such as comfort and ease of use, even if it the age-old folding massage table pattern, which has a skirt hiding legs that can be altered to suit different height requirements.

There are also massage tables available for extra storage and some even come with side-trays and lighting fixture scope so these can be closed down when not in use and store oils, sponges, cloths and incense etc. out of view and safely, but handy if needed.

The typical table-tops measure 30 inches wide and 76 inches in length; they have rounded corners so covers are easy to put on and no sharp edges protrude when the massage expert has to stretch across a client. Most good quality massage tables come with an added foam-insert that has a built-in face hole and padded table skirts so no hardware is apparently sticking out. Usually, they also have easily adjustable legs that can be operated with one knob and have

Massage Therapy For Complete Body Relaxation

center support braces to hold every part in place, held together by steel cables that do not allow the massage table to collapse under weight.

One can go in for the DIY type also and put together various locks, levers, knobs and screws to assemble the massage table of their requirement by following simple instructions, but this was mostly for the older version (with airplane wings that folded for easy storage and locked tight when in use). This variety cut back on using wood on the supports or legs to curtail weight, but all massage tables – whatever the pattern – do use generous amount of padding and plastic washers so the session is comfortable and peaceful.

If keen on one with wooden parts, check to see these are all curved nicely, sanded down and finished proper to give the surface an elegant look and remain snag-free; opting for the new soft feeling, tough-acting vinyl is a good idea for your massage table investment because it can stand up to a lot of wear and tear subject to body oils, sweat and toxins etc. besides being easy to clean.

So, go for quality (perhaps even add in the neck and leg pillow for added pampering) and choose a massage table that offers more facilities and rub up someone the right way!

Massage Chairs

Having an excellent health is top priority. This can be hard to achieve especially with daily work stress and time constrains. Not to mention going to have a relaxing day at the spa can be torture to your budget.

Among the relaxing benefits of having a good massage is loosening up of tight tissues in the body that will improve the flow of blood in the system. When blood flows smoothly it helps the regeneration of new skin cells and flashes out toxins in the body more efficiently. Exercise can be another way to do this, but it can prove to e taxing to do. This is way more and more people tend to have relaxing massages instead.

Because busy schedules we tend to postpone going to the massage spas to have our body taken cared of. That's why a large number of massagers are now available in the market today. They vary in functionality and look. But one of the most sot after is the chair massager.

The next impediment of having these relaxation machinery is that they are expensive to have. Yet, come to think about it you will only have to buy it once. Then soon after that, it will be with you for a lifetime. A good investment for your well deserved tired body.

If there is a brewing wish to buy one, know a couple or so specifics about it first.

- **Functionality**

Before buying anything, first be as critical as you can be. This will make your choice easier to come by. Know the count of kneading mechanism on the chair. Then, ask about how they function on the body.

- **Comfort**

Try out the chair! Be receptive on the comfort ability of the massage chair. Ask for padding and other footrest adjustability.

- **Operation**

Take the machine on a test ride on your body. This will ensure the way the machine will knead, tap and roll on muscles areas giving you more or less what to expect. Ask the operating attendant about how those manipulation rollers are built. If they are individually installed with separate motors, they will surely last longer. This massager may cost a little more than the single motor. Don't get too excited with massage chairs that offer lots of rollers, this will not immediately follow that they perform better. The important thing to keep in mind is to get one that has separate motors running them.

- **Controls**

Never forget to get in-depth information on all the aspects of the massage chair. One of the most essential queries is pressure adjustments. The control of the rollers needs to have the capacity to go fast, put more pressure or reduce pressure for a softer massage experience. Never forget to take into account the flexibility of the chair as it adjusts to different body types.

- **Price**

This is the question that begs to get the right answer, how much? Depending on the performance and the holistic feature of the massage chair, the price will definitely vary. They range from eight hundred USD to four thousand USD. Reputation of the store from which you're going to buy your massager from is a good start when hunting. Online shopping is also an alternative way to get a hold of good products. Be reminded of a return policy that comes with the merchandise, particularly when buying online. This will make sure that if you are not satisfied with it you will be able to send it back to the manufacturer or store you bought it from. Also is good when it is broken or has malfunctioned, being protected by a return policy will keep your purchase secure. Warranties are another important consideration. If they have a lifetime warranty, even if it is more expensive you will be shielded for years to come each time the massager breaks down.

<u>Massage Oils</u>

As far back as the ancient times dating even farther than the Egyptian civilization, oil has been used by man. It has demonstrated its powers in varied ways. The usefulness of oil from food, medicine and beauty products proves it has no bound on its impact in our live.

In this generation, in particular, when everyone is too caught up in spawning financial glory stress levels are sky high. Oil comes into play as an ally to help ease anxiety though oil massages and medicinal products, which has been establish well by scholars in the past dating back to 1000 B.C.

Oil products come from nature mostly in plant seeds, roots, bark, flowers and leaves. Elemental in nature they are called essential oils. Different characteristics of plants give distinct smell, flavor and effect for application. To name a few are safflower for blood purifier (easily turns sour), almond oil to minimize swelling and olive oil loosen stiff muscles. Other properties of oil are antifungal or antibacterial. Yet on the lighter side they are also used for aroma therapy, which heals the well being and emotional state.

Smooth, soft, younger looking and moisturized skin is very woman's desire. Castor oil can leave your skin scar free. Vitamins A and E are extracted from avocado and can be used by all types of skin for nourishment. For those stubborn pimples jojoba oil is the best bet. It combats oily secretion of skin pores to a least possible degree.

As a recreational substance oils are used for sensual massages. The greasy trait in it allows the masseuse's slithering hands to effortlessly penetrate the body's pressure points . Though this may be good for the masseuse it is frowned upon by the person on the massage table. That's why there are light oils that don't leave heavy grease on the body.

Aroma therapy was mentioned earlier. The combination of aroma stimulant and soothing rubdown can send the senses wild. Two of which are oil based. Spas are banking on the mood like deem lights, music and enticing atmosphere to bring tranquility to their customers. They are never with out oil based products to elicit a serene indulgence.

Massage Therapy For Complete Body Relaxation

Additives boost oil to exploit its effectiveness. Aloe Vera when added to oil restores irritated and bunt skin. For blood flow can be improved with adding cayenne to oil. Extracts form grape seeds acts as antibacterial to kill viruses dodging infections away from the body. But never use or put on oil where there is an open wound involve. This may do more harm than good.

As a responsible consumer, always check the labels for information on the oil based products you're about to buy. Knowing the substance can help you avoid allergic reactions that can put your health at risk. Be reminded of application instructions and cautionary directions on the labels.

Storage information is also a key player to extend the life of oil based products. Spoilage rate increases with high oxidation rate. Drops of Vitamin E can preserve your massage oil month after month. Usually, it stay longer if they were not subjected in too much high temperature while being processed. So it is well advice to watch out for words like cold-pressed or expeller-pressed. Refrigerate your oil products avoid premature or rapid decay.

Looking after your health is the most important aspect of living. Make sure to double check your allergens by consulting your doctor first before using any products.

Asian Massage – 5 Best Ways To Relieve Stress!

The power and peacefulness of being able to relax after an Asian Massage session is to experience in person in order for anyone to know how invigorating and stress-relieving it can be at the same time.

While Asia has long been regarded as the home for varied cultural and alternate healthcare practices that combine the elements of agony, ecstasy, higher knowledge and consciousness besides being enjoyable, stress-relieving and also strengthening – both physically and mentally, not many people know of the 5 basic Asian massage forms and their benefits. We cover some of these proven techniques and their advantages for the reader interested in balancing the energies of the body and mind through the best relaxation techniques man has ever know i.e. Asian Massage.

There are many different types of massages in the world, each with its own basic techniques and benefits for those who believe in taking up activities to nourish mind and body; among the most popular are Shiatsu, Acupressure, Amma (or anma), Ayurvedic and Champissage.

- **Shiatsu** – originated from Japan and focuses on using the fingers and acupuncture points for rewarding the person undergoing the massage a uniquely Oriental healing touch by controlling and balancing the flow of life energy that passes through the body. It concentrates in bringing about self-healing for the body through redirecting its own energies by applying slow pressure and stimulating blood flow, which in turn, brings about a sense of relief and relaxation besides also facilitating the human body's mechanism against disease of many kinds.
- **Acupressure** – is a Chinese technique for bringing rest from pain for the human body and focuses on using the fingers to press focal points on the body so tension and stress built up in the body is released and good sleep is ensured after the session. It is also a method for treating anxiety.
- **Anma (or Anma)** – is yet another Japanese healing technique, which means 'massage' in their language; it combines different limb movements to help a person experience peace and relief from pain and stress. It is based on the principles of a dance-like activity called Kata, which works to build up a tempo, pace and precision in the manner in which the masseuse decides different finger strokes, knee and elbow movements, stretching or

manipulating the feet and hands and thus, requires the body to be agile and flexible. Anma does not call for taking off one's clothes and can be practiced anywhere since no oils are used.

- **Ayurvedic** – is an Indian form of body massage used to cleanse the body of toxins and is based on vigorous hand strokes to bring about a sense of peacefulness and restore balance in the body. It typically uses warm oil and concoctions of herbs to get the right results and sometimes the massage oil is poured into the ears, between the brows and other specific energy points, with a client's permission.

- **Champissage**- has its root in Ayuveda; it is a technique that mainly deals with treating the upper half of the body in the aim of promoting blood circulation in the scalp. It nourishes the hair roots essentially but the feel-good feeling persists as the masseur also massages the client's face, neck, ears, neck and shoulders besides upper arms to get all the cricks out. It is believed to relieve headaches, eye-strain and energize a person.

Try one today – and feel lighter and more relaxed than ever before!

<u>Body Massage – Some Ground Rules For Building A Relationship</u>

There is a lot of truth in the old adage of seeing is believing; especially in a man-woman relationship, thoughtful actions do speak louder than words. So, what better way to show you care than expressing it through a caring and timely body massage treatment given to your partner? We show you how!

While typical men may think there's nothing better they'd like than having a wife's ministering touches, there is more to building intimacy in a relationship than simply love-making; yes, a massage is just as good as a hug that denotes all the love one feels without any undue pressure for sex. It is a joyful and stress-relieving activity that is highly recommended by experts who feel that building a relationship requires trust and to generate that in a woman, a man must learn techniques that make her feel relaxed, at ease with him and her body without any sexual advances feared.

The importance of a massage cannot be stressed enough in a loving relationship as the smallest tactile movements enable a child to know safety in a mothers' arms, so the lover feels warm and cherished when treated to tender and nourishing body massage that stretches the single touch to many more. Many women may have been physically abused in the past or suffered a recent trauma or just be basically shy to invite a massage readily but it is up to the man in her life to convince her of his intentions in wanting to do something special for she is special – and out of the bed, too.

The first step is to make a woman feel comfortable in your presence and help her relax so she is certain it will lead to bigger things; this is especially important for women with a troubled past who can end up losing out on their trust if pressed into sexual intimacy after a massage session for the sake of it.

Do it without expecting payment in kind and convince your woman it is for her sake that you are offering the body massage and while it is likely you will be aroused by the activity, clothe yourself properly to avoid showing any signs of the same.

Massage Therapy For Complete Body Relaxation

You can begin by preparing a bath for your woman, then lying her down on a clean towel or soft blanket on the floor instead of a bed, since the surface of a massage point needs to be firm. Put a pillow each below her head and shins and if you are not using pre-warmed, lightly-scented oil; you can cup some in your hands to transfer some body-heat to it before you begin by working on her shoulders and down her back, using slow strokes.

Pay close attention to any body parts that feel tense or stiff to your touch and ask where she hurts (if applicable) and work on those especially before moving to her thighs, legs and feet that need to be worked in circular motions before repeating the movements upwards again.

Avoid massaging private parts as you want her to relax and do not stare; work on her breasts only upon being given permission. Massage hands and face with a gentle touch and let her know in words how special she is – restrain your own needs, let it be her day, today!

<u>Breast Massage – Benefits Of Loving Your Body!</u>

Many women feel that they need to be dressed to kill in order to look good, but this is what many fancy garments may just as well be – for market research reveals that tight, constricting clothing and ill-chosen undergarments can be a primary cause for promoting breast cancer. We recommend breast massage for staying on top of things!

The reason why the current fascination for breast massage has gained so much attention is due to the fact that experts believe that wearing restrictive clothing that decompresses or enhances body parts such as whale-bone bras and corsets besides tummy-trimmer panties is because the emphasis on over-shapeliness causes toxins in the body to accumulate, whereas they need to be released from the tissues. When these are not flushed out properly and regularly, it can lead to unhealthy levels of toxicity in the breast tissues and eventually to breast cancer.

However, experts also recommend that since this is one of the reasons for promoting breast cancer, it is better to focus on the preventive nature of the same and raise awareness about ways to educate women we love about avoiding the condition altogether – and so we have medical experts advocating regular breast massages as a preventive step for breast cancer.

The argument stems from the belief that the increased blood circulation caused by breast massage builds up to a warmth suffusing the breast area that works to flush-out toxin from this delicate zone besides encouraging the lymph fluids to flow easily so they help in draining out remaining chemicals that may be harmful. (The lymph fluids are the watery liquid surrounding the cells; they contain disease-fighting components and thus are important to pay attention to in cases of a family history of breast cancer or for those at risk for it).

A breast massage is very beneficial for women and it can be practiced on self or by someone else. It requires a gentle kneading movement combined with rubbing or squeezing techniques to induce improved blood and lymph flow; it is best done by gently stroking in a circular direction from the nipple out to the breast outline. Repeat the step a few times like you would if you ran your fingers along wheel-spokes – but avoid any aggressive stroking as this can be harmful.

You may use scented lotions or warm massage oils to build up the pleasure of the breast massage and to prevent any hand-rubbing friction caused in the lack of these 'helpers.'

Massage Therapy For Complete Body Relaxation

Ideally, breast massages should be performed at the end of a working day when shedding clothes and it is also recommend that women do not wear their bra and sleep (no more than 12hrs).

Other times a breast massage helps are when during a premenstrual cycle when some women suffer tenderness in their breasts; during nursing after surgery to reduce scar tissue marks and simply as an activity that keeps them a-breast with their bodily changes (such as a lump in the breast), which is easy to notice for those that regularly breast massage.

Erotic Massage

Everyone knows that variety is the spice of life but since safe sex is recommend for a healthy life and relationship management even if morality doesn't quite hold up the argument, the best thing to do to add excitement – minus the dangers of unprotected intercourse - to your intimate life is to learn the techniques of erotic massage!

One needn't be an expert in giving massages to experience the pleasure of innovating on some basic techniques to elicit the same pleasure in their partner and erotic massages are more than simply learning the right hand movements or a single touch: it's an art that needs to be built upon.

Learning the techniques of an erotic massage can also help people in overcoming the dissatisfaction that creeps in to many sexual relationships and hangs over like a shadow into their personal and professional lives as it leaves individuals feeling discontented and disenchanted with a segment of their lives that should be open to experimenting and excitement.

Besides bringing in a certain lost charm about their own sexuality, an erotic massage can help a person practice touches on themselves without the need for telling a partner how and where to touch for how long and re-connect with their bodily needs at their own leisure, for their own pleasure! It is recommended for both men and women with strong needs and desires and all that is called for is creating the right ambience and having an open mind to enjoying the beauty of the human body.

An erotic massage given right and accepted in the right mind can lead to a foreign thrill that is orgasmic in the joy it provides besides helping one relax independently, or with a partner (should one choose to share the knowledge). One doesn't even need an external stimulator for performing an erotic massage and it is as pleasurable in giving one as receiving one – so try it today!

A flat, firm surface is needed for performing an erotic massage and touches need to be intimate, warm and sensual to build up to a crescendo within the individual's body and bring about utter

Massage Therapy For Complete Body Relaxation

peace and ultimate relaxation from the session. When concentrating on the person's sexual points, it is advisable to keep the tempo going and steady at a plateau of feelings before letting them experience the high of the ultimate arousal.

Men like being spoken to during the erotic massage but many may react just as well to non-verbal strokes to bring them to ejaculate while women are more given towards receiving erotic massage when it concentrates on their G-Spot (also known as the clitoral massage), which if done properly, can bring them to multiple orgasms.

An erotic massage can be performed for opposite sex or same-sex partners and be equally stimulating in either case but remember, there is little room for selfishness and wanting to satisfy your own urges when conducting an erotic massage – so, learn to give pleasure in order to be the best lover you can be!

Male Massage

Male massages are primary a massage session between a client and a male masseur and are rising in popularity with the number of parlors opening up around the globe only catering to specific demands for these experts with magic hands. It is believed that a man's strong and capable hands are better suited to releasing tension from various bodily parts and thus better at relieving stress.

A massage may well have been looked upon as something that was woman-pleasure oriented or meant for the gay community, but with the evolution of the metro-sexual urban male who believes in looking good and feeling good in every sense, there is an acceptance about straight men of all ages visiting massage parlors for knocking some of the knots out of their system. Not only does a massage help work on stressed muscles and promote blood circulation, it also helps a man relax and free the day's tensions from his mind and body by helping the client achieve a sense of balance and peace through using stronger and effective techniques for inducing sleep, the ultimate relaxant.

A masseuse is a woman who though be well-trained in the various forms of massages or specializing in one particular form, but she is physically less likely to have the basic strength of men, who are more capable on the whole of exerting the strength and pressure needed on various joints in a man's body to rid him of the cricks than a woman massage expert ever could. Of course, we are not talking of the Swedish masseuse, but rather, women masseuse in general! Some men like a male massage expert working on them because of the added muscle power at their disposal so they are likely to get the tight knots of tension out of their system faster, others may prefer it as a fantasy-mode thing – especially gay men who enjoy it more due to associating it with a lover's touch.

Yes, there are homosexual masseurs as well as straight masseurs who service the otherwise inclined or straight lot of male clients in the various top-class as well as budget massage parlors that have sprung up in many tourist spots besides those that offer fringe benefits such as erotic massages or more intimate touching to the clients.

Many men come back to the male massage parlors for the choice of a sensual massage as they are allowed to build on the freedom and willingness of the masseur, but others are quite strict

Massage Therapy For Complete Body Relaxation

about the kind of services offered being only restricted to non-sensual relaxation techniques. Moreover, depending on the parlor one chooses, one may be required to shed their clothes or keep them on while the thrill factor for some parlors comes with some masseurs even working nude!

You can have a private massage session at home or go to a hotel, but the right ambience is necessary to get the right results of pleasure and relaxation from a perfect massage, so choose what you are comfortable with. And if all else fails, you can build up your own skills at massaging and exchange one with your partner!

<u>Las Vegas Massage Therapy</u>

Surfeit of fun and enjoyment is the key essence of all activities in Las Vegas. As such, Las Vegas massage therapy is just an extension of the principle of living or playing in fun in Las Vegas. Both the residents and visitors to Las Vegas have a lot of choices when it comes to massage therapy.

Options and locations for Las Vegas Massage Therapy are virtually unlimited. A Las Vegas massage therapist can always be found close at hand, for anybody keen on getting massage therapy done. Health as well as relaxation being the focus of visitors, massage therapists in Las Vegas come with different settings to deliver the desired services, in a comfortable and fun location.

Obviously, there are a large number of spas, casinos, hotels and resorts of all categories in Las Vegas. All of them have a facility for massage therapy as all of them are focused on relaxation and pleasure of their visitors. People come to Las Vegas for rejuvenation and stress relief, so the vacations are designed to be relaxing. Massage therapists use numerous massage techniques or styles, each having a distinct advantage for the customer, according to their individual physical and health characteristics.

In a resort location, massage therapy services maybe made available in a massage office or in the hotel room where the person is staying. There are also mobile massage therapists, offering the choice of private massage to both the residents of Las Vegas as well as to the visitors. Mobile massage therapists make sure that you never need to leave your room, for the sake of a massage.

Local advertisements, search on the internet, referral by physicians or the staff at spas/ hotels, location services of associations like the American Massage Therapy Association and word of mouth references can all help you get in touch with mobile massage therapists.

Las Vegas massage therapy is beneficial not just for the visitors but also for the people living and working in Las Vegas. Problems like stress and muscle tension affect all and every body can benefit from improved circulation and fluid joints. Also, sports related injuries may be healed

Massage Therapy For Complete Body Relaxation

and performance in athletics can also be enhanced with Las Vegas massage therapy. For the resident clients, not just mobile massage therapists, but other options to get professional Las Vegas massage therapy will just as well.

Las Vegas massage therapy services for managing health can be accessed at the medical centers of physicians, private offices for massage therapy, sports facilities and clinics offering sports medicine, health centers, chiropractic offices, gyms and fitness centers.

Las Vegas massage therapy service is available to anybody that needs it or just has a desire to relax, from any number of easily accessible and professionally qualified massage therapists.

Austin School Of Massage Therapy

Studying to have a good living is the best way to make something out your life. One of the more popular studies nowadays is therapeutic massaging. This article talks about a certain school that can offer this.

Therapeutic Massages in the U.S. are in demand. Plenty of students want to study there. But the most popular of them all is the Austin School of Massage Therapy located in Texas.

What's in this Institute of Massage Therapy:

ASM produces a good quality graduates in therapy for 25 years. Recognition was given to them as the most productive school for therapy. The school has 8000 graduates and become popular and in demand profession in U.S.

It is being recognize internationally and increase its production and name as the biggest massage therapy in that country. Modern program for students are being introduced to insure that they choose the right profession. The have tested and successfully achieved the credit of a good standard. **ASMT offers the following program for students**.

- Class Venue
- Offer specialization Program (to give reasonable salary as incentives as high as $75.00 an hour) including maternity care, child birth, baby massage, body and foot spa massage and even in medical and palliative care management program. Certificate of Attendance are given to anybody including private practitioner as long as they participate on this program.
- Offer comprehensive program for 500 hours non stop.
- Free tuition to those who are qualified to be a scholar.
- The Massage therapy store that carries supplies is open for 24 hours.

 The ASMT continue to support their program. They provide a good assistance and better job opportunities to their graduates. The school maintains high standard of education to help graduates pass the licensure examination and help graduates to improved their knowledge about modern technology.

Massage Therapy For Complete Body Relaxation

A.S.M.T.– Expansion program

Austin has able to expand the outreach program throughout the U.S. There are 12 branches that almost open and operates within Texas alone. Most students select to which key metropolis in the Lone Star state they can enroll themselves for they have the same goal, to provide productive graduates.

In addition to this, students and some residents can avail and can schedule a massage session. Advertisements and some form of information are being disseminated to the public in order to inform them about their purpose. This will help them in honing their skills further.

As being known to be the most popular school for massage therapy they have expanded in the whole of the U.S. Plaque of Appreciation and Recognition are being awarded to them for a job well done, and as best school in Texas. Happy to say the help find job for their graduates and provide good education to those who are interested.

Doing The Back Massage – Doing It The Best Way

Back massages are one of the most common and loved massages of all time. Lean the ways to do it so that you can give it to your loved ones at home.

Back massages are just one of the amazing experiences there is that will surely take your stress off your body. There is a huge part of our time spent earning and become our into dream life. Every moment of the day, it is all about work and other people before ourselves. We feel its toll by the time our temper changes and we become a walking time bomb. Shortly after this work becomes stressful, leaving us to feel burnt-out. Physical tiredness can be observed when our posture starts to be imbalanced.

The benefits of the getting a back massage weighs more than not having one. Not only does it promote total relaxation it does wonders to your health too. For starters, it improves blood circulation. This implies lesser strain on the whole body. The lymphatic drainage is better with filtering toxins.

So, there is one thing left to do know how to give properly. First, as the name suggest it should be done on the back. This means that the one to be massaged should lie on their belly which is very comfortable and smooth. Use foam or a cushion to make relaxing blissful. Protect your back as well by making sure that the height of the massage table or bed is just right. If it's too low then this will make your back pain and injure you along the way. If it is too high, the pressure that you need to place on the back might be lesser that what is necessary. As you are standing or kneeling at the bed or floor side rub your hands to make it warm before doing anything. Then place your hands on the edge of the shoulder blades, over the heart and the other on the lower part of the back.

The back is loosen up by placing pressure down the spine's sides starting from the lower back to the neck. While doing this use your thumb and press in circular motion as you trace the spine's sides. Effleurage, minor strokes, can be applied to add variation to the rubdown as you level down the oil or lotion on the back. With one long constant stroke slide your palms entirely down both side of the pelvis; scrape from hips and reverse up the surface to the shoulder. To start on a fresh spot, travel your hands easily on the back. Continue on equally on the neck base.

Massage Therapy For Complete Body Relaxation

Begin at the spine and slither your palms in opposing courses going outwards to the edges of the back. Beginning at the back's lowers portion then move up to the shoulders. Softly rub the plump muscular section at the peak of the shoulders, the back's middle portion as well as the buttocks to loosen off stiff connective tissues or fascia and muscles. Place pressure on the tense region of the back, also known as knot, massaging it with the palms or fingers. Carry out clockwise resistance in circular motion with the tips of your fingers through the muscles which are confined to the spine plus the area of the shoulder blades. Move out the arms around it gently, individually, uniting the joints in the shoulder, which adds to better circulation of the blood.

With this kind of technique the benefits are good. It allows wellness of the mental state in account of relaxation. The feeling of rejuvenation is carried out along the full back's tight muscles. It lets the tissues that have been tightened for a long time slacken, in turn gives way for the flow of blood to become continuous. This massage is best done with lubricating liquids to minimize friction during the rubdown session. It can be between the choice of a lotion or an oil essential with a relaxing aromatic smell.

Foot Massage - 6 Excellent Ways To Pamper Your Feet

This article will help you through instructions on how to get a quick and easy foot massage. It aims to help you achieve a happy feet.

There are a lot of different massages that target different parts of the body. The most satisfying of them is a foot massage. Reason behind it is that the feet are the most worked of our external body organ. They carry around body weight whether standing or on the move. Thus, pampering it will give unspeakable pleasure as stress is being rid from it. Blood circulation will be improved as muscles relax during massage.

Relaxing the feet with massages is also believed to be beneficial to the whole body. By using different degrees of pressure at specific areas on it yield endorphins. These chemicals are natural pain killers that help the body from tensing up. Just the right pressure on the feet intervenes with diseases from progressing.

Getting started on your feet is easy enough. It can be done with the use of oil essentials, foot lotions or any other form of lubricant. Doing it with someone else can bring sheer delight, although you can also manage on your own. Best be sitting on the most relaxing chair to insure your back is properly supported if you are lacking helping hands to massage for you. A chair that has an arm rest cushion and footrest will do the trick. Now you can start the massage by placing on your lap on foot then do these simple steps. Soon enough you'll find yourself smiling and your feet happy at last.

1.   **Top to bottom rub**

Generating heat is the first agenda to relax and fill-up the feet. Begin working from the top rubbing your way down use your thumb. Go up and down with one constant stroke from toes to your ankles. Do it over and over again for a few minutes.

2.   **Ankle twirling stokes**

Relaxing your toes as you give it a careful spin! This simple calisthenics does magic to those cramps on your joints. Continue by clamping on the foot as you gently turn it clockwise and counter clockwise for at least 4-5 times respectively. Remember that any sudden rotation of the ankles can cause unsolicited injuries. The idea is to relieve stress from your feet, not the other way around.

3.   **Pin it down with pressure**

Now that the foot is prep for the main massage, hold it closely with the other hand and use the other to place pressure to it. Then pin down the thumb gently starting with the biggest toes on the soles in 2-4 counts. Then release the pressure soothingly working your way through the next toe. When pinning down, reel the thumb in and out. Then complete this step by varying the degrees of pressure applied on the foot's surface.

4.   **Press at leisurely pace**

From smaller areas that are pinned down, go wider by the use of knuckles. This time bigger spaces are reached all at once, giving a different sensation of relaxation, not only for the foot but for the whole body as well.

5.   **Slither fingers amid the toes**

In a rhythmic motion reach in between the toes using the fingers to exercise and relax the tense muscles of the toes. Do a back and forth fluid motion to pamper those over worked toes.

6.   **Press the sole's depression**

Push the depression of the foot very hard using the knuckles or heels of the hand. Relief will come as soon as the inner and outer curve of the foot's sole releases the pressure. Squeeze the entire foot hard enough to create a soothing finish to this relaxing massage. Before wrapping-up to a close, make sure not to leave out anything unmassaged like the sides, top, bottom and everything in between it.

If you're being assisted by someone else on this relaxing rubdown, make sure to tell them how much pressure you can tolerate. Anything that causes unbearable pain in a massage must alarm you to stop and have it taken a look by a doctor.

The feet work hard. It deserves to at least have a happy hour after working. Therefore, good relaxing massages makes for happy feet.

Swedish Massage

Swedish massage's a technique used by masseuse to help the body in timing-out from its pressure driven existence. Get to know this method better so that you'll be able to request it when you get to have a body massage done on your weary body.

Detoxifying the body after a lengthy workday can bring you to a better place of de-stressing into wellness. As a very popular choice, the Swedish massage has been in use for so many years by masseuse in the west. It doesn't only focuses on one area of the body it certainly is a total body massage. It massages from head to toe.

First came into being in Sweden by a man named Pen Henrik Ling in the year 1830. Its name spread throughout the massage world employing variations of pressure to help with blood circulation. It intends to relax and loosen muscles by applying force ranging from gentle to hard as it stimulates the nerves endings while continuously rubbing the skin in the same course were blood flows to pump it back into the system.

This is manipulated by using extensive strokes, creating resistance and kneading on the top portion of muscles. These motions are use to bring the lost energy to the body avoiding blood clots that causes strokes and other ill effects. It helps the heart from strenuous toil that stress and blockage from circulation creates.

It is quite understandable to have apprehensions of getting this body massage because it must be done in nude. But, one needs to be informed that towels are used to conceal the privates and sensitive area of the body. This is important for masseuse to maintain the trust of their clients to create a longer business relationship.

Since this total body massage benefits more and more people its demand has reached a pinnacle of success. Masseuses all over different parts of the world are now studying this technique over another method. Reason being is that it has proven its value ability to the health community in terms remedial alternatives goes.

As an aesthetic means for enhancing the skin it can smoothen and scrub down dead skin cells. When the masseuse uses a pebbly lotion, this can help rough skin from thinning. As it is

Massage Therapy For Complete Body Relaxation

thoroughly stroked deeper into the skin, it leaves a fresh layer to glow after. As a result a baby soft smooth skin is revealed.

For those who are having issues with cellulite, this total body massage adds more flexibility to the muscles and skin tissues. Those stubborn calcified fats trapped on the skin are slowly liberated. But, don't expect it to immediately go away in one session. This can be achieved in many follow-ups, which is constantly kept. For those who would like to accomplish toner skin after losing a lot of weight this can also be made possible by this massage. It flexes the skin and promotes better elasticity. There are some masseuses who claim that a total body massage can reach small muscle groups that are not used frequently toning them better than any exercise compared.

If exercising can help those muscles bulk up and tighten, massaging will make them loose and tone. They can both be good for the health, yet comparatively massages are more favored by people who wants to have a healthy life at the same time brings serenity. With all the noise and toxins that the body receives everyday it is an essential practice to let it all out. Swedish massage can help you flush out those unwanted dirt in the body.

Bare Naked Massage

In line with massages, being nude is part of experiencing total relaxation with a touch and warm hands. This let you see how it can be satisfying to the senses and stress relieving to the nerves.

Awakening your nerve endings gives you an instant sensual change. Anybody can show their emotions in so many ways. Eye contact, an erotic smile, or a sweet whisper in the car. While we experiment on the feeling of how nude massage is, it would be much appreciated and exciting if you do it with someone you feel attracted to. Go ahead it will give you a pleasant day after a hard day of work.

At first this kind of massage is a little awkward to both of you. It takes a minute for both of you to get comfortable to it. Surely you will expect something special and memorable if you ease to it. It is not only a part of a game or fling with somebody else. Sometimes it becomes a regular ritual to both of you.

Nude massage need some extra attention like what kind of place are you going to take. Is it suitable for both lovers? Should you lose your self esteem or develop self confidence.

Massage oil is a big factor that can contribute to this. Select the best one that can penetrate deeply in your skin, and the aroma of it. Smell the goodness of the oil while starting the nude massage unconsciously both of you start to enjoy and feel a deeper feeling with each other. Lust and ambivalent feelings are being thrown out in the open. Who knows, it may eventually develop into something more special in the future.

A warm light or better yet, scented candle is more romantic. Choose one which has a mild but exotic smell that can relax your nerves and both of you will enjoy what you have started.

A romantic and conducive place to both lovers is the one of the most important factor in nude massage. Sometimes a glass of wine and soft music playing on the background contributes a slow rhythm in the first part of the massage session. You should know there are better ways of giving a boost to your confidence and nude massage is one of them.

Massage Therapy For Complete Body Relaxation

All set for a romantic massage

(getting started on the massage in nude)

Prepare yourself by applying some sweet scented lotion oil in your neck and start a mild massage to ease the fear. Rubbing your neck and shoulders, releases stress. Better wear a towel or being half nude is okay too. It makes you look more appealing. Be positive by having a special moment with your partner who is worth remembering. Prepare yourself to start the nude massage session. Relax.

Position your partner in bed either back lying or other positive that suits her or him. See to it that it's a relaxing position. Start rubbing over the neck from the back of the head in a very soft and mild stroke using your palm. Mild strokes will do no harm. It helps to relax muscles and ease back pain. It contributes a sensual feeling in your partner. To intensify your touch, give some frisky nips to the neck, abdomen, and thighs.

Many people erroneously believe that to be happy as partners, you need to be having frequent, spontaneous love making through making them feel wanted and loved. Do not be in a hurry and take your extra time in doing the back rubbing every so often. It will be exciting to both of you.

Also keep in mind what you are doing is one way of combining both feelings of excitement. Allow your hands to tease the nape of your partner's neck. Be gentle and the heat of the oil relaxes your muscle, heightens skin sensation which causes you to slow down and get in touch with your partner.

Give a smooth stroke on the thigh, legs and feet. There's nothing more exciting than the smell and the soft touch of your palm. Then send your partner into a foreplay frenzy by massaging the body with your own. With your vivid imagination, apply a firm manhandling to let him become turned on and have his pleasure pushed to the next level of love making.

You can make the most of this effect by taking sweet time together and frankly speaking its quiet remembering.`

Prostate Massage

Sex is not a subject for the lighthearted. You need a bit more courage to talk about it openly. You may if not for media and all the freedom of speech in the world people will never get the courage to conquer their inhibitions about the subject. Surprisingly, society has slowly gotten to that point. Women talk about the long-ago taboos amongst themselves, usually they love to discuss the many ways they are not getting pleasure out of having sex and exchange notes on improving their performance in bed. It seems that any dinner get together among close friends in no way ends without touching base on this subject. Probably those years of suppression of the topic catches-up to it now.

Men are the shy ones to speak openly about sex in a more serious tone. They usually use it as anecdotes and sarcastic comments to express their undeclared sentiments on the matter. Believe it or not, pleasuring man doesn't only start and stop when they get off. There are other ways to give them satisfaction.

If you're looking for ways give him an ultimate bedtime loving, here is a new technique for you. The massaging the prostate is the new word that not only pleasures him but also has health benefits.

There are reservations about this massage. One question that begs an answers is how can it bring pleasure? G-spot it the ultimate answer to this. This is a part of the males genitals that has the highest concentration of small nerves. When touched or rubbed they create sensations that bring pleasure. If the massage is done correctly, this will liberate enormous amount of satisfaction and helps relax the body as it surrenders to it completely. As the body relaxes, stress is discharged from it. When this massage when concurrent with stroking the penis gives an explosive pleasure for men.

Apart from intensifying his ejaculation response sensation, this massage furthermore amplifies anal feeling, resulting to an unforgettable experience. On of the hugely gratifying effects of the prostate rubdown is it facilitates the unseen penis within the body to get satisfaction simultaneously with the prostate. The upshot of this stimulation as a threesome is breathtaking. Nevertheless, more grander in effect by the physical aspect is its impact to the psychological

Massage Therapy For Complete Body Relaxation

facet of the man's psyche. This can be accounted for due to the act of penetration, which unfamiliar to the man's body.

Apart from enlightening the body to a new experience, massively this massage will create a "cerebral high", it is also used to cater to the health needs of the anal as well. This can be done without the help of a partner. All that needs to be done is to simply place in a finger or two into the anal canal reaching flipside and upwards in the direction of the navel in anticipation of the prostate gland. Still, it will bring more enjoyment if there is a partner to share it with. Climax will come easily with having less hesitation and a lot of confidence in the execution of this erotic act.

Homosexuality is a big misconception on people who are going the prostate therapeutic massage. Because this is a very sensitive area this particular massage are done by couples in the privacy of their bedrooms. Yet, study show that this massage is essential for men to prevent future complications in the prostate areas. Doctors have given this as a prescribed massage for men who have illnesses that affect their prostate. But, unfortunately fear get the better of them, that's why it is quite a taboo for straight men to have one with their partners. The lack of working-out the prostate can head toward dysfunction, malfunction and other prostate diseases.

There is no known study that will prove men turning homosexuals just because they were exercising their prostate gland. But, doctors will tell you your health is in grave danger if you do not do it.

The Art Of Sensual Massage

Partners that are in a longtime relationship are sometimes tired of their old routines. There is a good way to spice up the connection between then in the bedroom. The sensual massage can help them liven up again.

There are many things that most couples enjoy doing together on their free time. They can go to malls and watch a movie. Then probably afterwards they have dinner and wine. But, when the blinds are closed intimacy then starts to brew. A good way to end the date is through a sensual massage. This is conducive for couples who are very comfortable with their sexuality.

The most sensitive and enjoyable massage is the sensual one. It creates mutual feeling and understanding to both partners. Set the day right. Observe what kind of partner you go with. Younger ones are fond of touching and experiencing this kind of massage.

There are different kinds of approaching and applying this form of massage. Medical experts apply sensual massage in a part of body where harm had been damaged. It could be good. Back massage can release stress. Sensual massage can lead to intimacy to both partners. Touching ones body create a sensitive sensation.

The feeling aroused is the unusual chilling sensation your body get. It turns into an extra warm feeling making you hypersensitive, that little by little your pleasure points are exploding in every minute they are touched, leaving you only a feeling of an ultra lusty rush. Sensual massage relaxes your muscles, heightens skin sensation and enhances your overall experience. There is no reason to restrain yourself from this massage if that someone is a person you genuinely care about. Massages are good rubdowns which makes one passionate relationship.

Always tell your partner that at the moment you should practice modern massage and leave behind old time massage. Let it start a mild one until the time your partner responds to build a closer relation with each other. Time can tell that both of you have the sensuous feeling emotionally to experience.

Always discuss with your partner the right spot in your body that makes your feel most sensual when touched. This will make the two of you reminisce about why you're together. when time

Massage Therapy For Complete Body Relaxation

comes for the actual massage, don't just do the usually practiced old way of massaging. This time try to introduce and fuse a more modern method. Initiate a good tactic by starting the massage at the nape of the neck and slowly going down the body until the feeling of eagerness and excitement starts. The whole thing follows. Enjoy a night of wonderful and exotic music while performing the sensual massage.

You can imagine if both of you enjoy this kind of massage. First make sure the place is quiet. Light up an aromatic set of scented candles around the place the smell of will help you get in the mood faster. A good romantic music can do the trick as well. Make sure the place , the bed sheets and the pillow cases are clean smelling fresh. Place some rose petals around the bed or on it to conjure a romantic atmosphere.

A good hot bath is highly recommended before starting on anything, to take away some dirt from your body. You can both take the bath together to lure the mood in. You should keep in mind that the process of a good sensual massage will only be a success when both partners can touch each other. Equally and mutually as the desire to give and take pleasure must be the main goal.

You will notice that after the session, both partner have something in common that is enjoyment and a lifetime of happiness. Intimacy is very important start sparks which will ultimately lead into love making. A good end of a sensual massage will give good memories that are a memorably unforgettable experience to both partner. Bring something into the bedroom that's new and exciting. Then you'll know that relaxing and satisfying sensual massage will keep the fire in your relationship burning.

Massage Therapy Careers

Massage therapy careers are becoming more and more popular day by day, due to heightened awareness, growing demand and general acceptance that massage therapy treatment is a key part of health management solutions. This in turn has led to increased opportunities for new graduates of massage therapy programs as well as for therapists having experience.

People in the know forecast a bright future for massage therapy careers. The United States Department of Labor, Bureau of Labor Statistics, has said that careers linked to the massage therapy field are set to grow at a faster rate than other careers. This rate of better than average growth is expected to continue till the year 2014. Opportunities in the massage therapy field include both part time and full time jobs. Nearly two –third of the massage therapists in the United States are supposed to be self employed, either working as contractors or running their own massage therapy centers.

Massage therapy careers differ according to the settings they are housed in that may be either public or private. Self employed massage therapists may opt for a salary, hourly rate or contractor arrangements. Massage therapists can work in any of a wide range of establishments that includes self-employed positions, salaried, hourly, and contractor arrangements, massage therapists can be found working in any of a wide range of establishments that include spas & health clinics, resorts & salons, offices of physicians and chiropractors, rehabilitation centers, hospitals, gyms & fitness centers, private houses, nursing homes, corporate offices and fitness centers, alternative health centers & yoga studios, airports, mall, universities and basically any place that people need to fix their health.

The nature of jobs linked to massage therapy are those of Physical therapist, a therapist's assistant, sports massage therapist, masseuse, mobile massage therapist, massage therapy instructor or teacher and massage therapist.

A career in the massage therapy field can be quite demanding, both physically as well as in the toll that it takes on personal life. In physical terms, the body of the massage therapist may feel the effects as the job of a therapist involves standing for long hours and exerting physically. Fatigue sets in due to having to stand for a long time. People using an incorrect technique could

Massage Therapy For Complete Body Relaxation

even sustain physical injuries. Therefore, following the right technique and correct scheduling of appointments, with time gaps between each, can solve these problems.

As the job is physically very strenuous for the therapist, most massage therapists are able to actually perform massages for only about thirty hours each week. The US Department of Labor in fact considers fifteen to thirty hours of therapy per week as a full time job. All the same, the therapist may have to spend additional time to complete related administrative tasks.

The personal toll that the massage therapy profession takes is because the services of massage therapists are asked for mostly in the time that is off from work for people. Evening and weekend appointments are quite common even though once a therapist has built a name for himself or herself, they may be able to schedule client appointments in normal working hours.

While being demanding, a massage therapy career can also be very rewarding. All the same, people who are willing to take up the challenge also get all the rewards.

<u>Massage Therapy Insurance</u>

There are several choices in massage therapy insurance. Selecting a suitable insurance plan is a must when starting the business, for a massage therapist.

While the regulations vary from state to state and it is not even legally compulsory for all massage therapists to have insurance, it is still important for the massage therapist to have insurance, in case they ever get into a financially difficult situation. There are no defined standards or massage therapy insurance due to variations in each state's regulations. There are definitely no set rates and the cost of insurance can greatly differ for each state. However, these are no excuses for not having insurance.

There are numerous types of massage therapy insurance. Liability is a huge worry for massage therapists. Still, liability insurance is not the only type of massage therapy insurance around. Several types of insurances have been created to assure the personal safety of massage therapists. While these are all optional, it is in the interest of the massage therapist to purchase these insurance. Some of the recommended massage therapy insurance plans are:
health insurance if it is not made available by the employer or the person is self employed; property insurance, one each for both the home and the office and specially important if the office is at home itself and clients are visiting the place; renters or lease insurance in case the office premises are rented. This insurance should cover the replacement cost of products and equipment.

Other insurances cover business, dental expenses, automobile (this is critical if the vehicle is used for mobile massage therapy), and disability insurance that provides for expenses, in case the therapist loses the ability to work.

The procedure for purchasing massage therapy insurance is fairly simple, whether buying for personal or professional reasons. There are local insurance agents who sell different types of insurance. While purchasing, the massage therapist should keep in mind that the local agent may offer very limited choices or policies that are of a very general nature. The cost may also be higher. The reason for all these is that the local agent may have very few clients in the massage therapy field. So the massage therapist will have to perforce buy the insurance policy on an individual basis.

Massage Therapy For Complete Body Relaxation

Purchasing massage therapy insurance from a professional organization works best for most massage therapists. Professional organizations deal with massage therapy associations. Therefore, they have the expertise and know exactly the kind of insurance required by a therapist, inclusive of the protections and limits that are needed. Professional organizations also have a large size and larger groups comprising of a number of buyers have better purchasing power. This leads to cheaper policies, if they are purchased from professional organizations.

The right type of massage therapy insurance assures both personal and professional security by accidents, whether related to therapy or for some other reason, do not put a stop to the earning power of the massage therapist.

Massage Treatment Intake Forms

Massage treatment intake forms play a critical role where both the client and the therapist are concerned. Massage treatment intake forms convey a wealth of useful information that provides the starting point for treatment.

Why Massage Treatment Intake Forms Are Required By Therapists

Massage treatment intake forms are what go into the client's file first; they are intended to supply the therapist with the necessary information that will enable him to treat you for you problem in a sound and careful manner.

All patients do not receive the same massage treatment. There are a number of things that can influence the extent/regularity of treatment that you get, including the degree and duration of each session. Now what seems appropriate for you may in fact lead to injury in another person with a particular problem. The **queries mentioned in the massage treatment intake form** are intended to enlighten the therapist regarding your:

a. Medical history
b. Present medical problems
c. Extent of motion
d. Purpose of treatment
e. Personal viewpoint concerning massage therapy (for instance, do you consider massage to be a practicable physical therapy or just a soothing, relaxing, indulgence?)

Moreover, massage treatment intake forms also list the elementary requirements like contact data as well as confidentiality disclosure.

The replies given by you against each of the queries listed in the form will reveal to the massage therapist which specific areas require greater focus, the type of massage that will work best for you and tend to make you feel more comfortable, and if any products, techniques, or stimulations are contraindicated where you are concerned because of your problem or allergy and such others.

Massage Therapy For Complete Body Relaxation

The objective of massage treatment intake form is certainly to make available a unique massage treatment experience with the best possible results.

What Queries Are Included?

Now, your massage treatment intake form should by no means be excessively intrusive, but some basics are required. The standard massage intake form generally will comprise of queries that inquire about:

1. Your address and contact data

2. Levels of stress

3. Strain

4. Headaches

5. Medical conditions like high blood pressure, diabetes, epilepsy, circulatory and cardiac conditions

6. Latest procedures or problems such as surgery, broken bones, pregnancy, back problems, tissue damage

7. Problems with pain like back pain, sensitive areas, numbness, pressures, or piercing pains

Furthermore, you will have the chance to inform the therapist by means of the massage treatment intake form what your particular area(s) of distress is (are) and in what way you think massage therapy will benefit you.

Your massage therapist just requires you to complete a massage treatment intake form before your initial appointment, and at regular intervals following ongoing treatment. With the help of the information supplied by you, the therapist develops a massage procedure especially for you in order that you attain whatever you set to accomplish from your personal massage treatment experience.

Massage Therapy For Complete Body Relaxation

This Product Is Brought To You By

DAVID A OSEI

9 781710 207309